...he paradox that meditating on sickness can lead us to recognize

...or of *The Accidental Anarchist*

...' James Lang writes, 'does not present itself . . . as an open ..., like everything we find in the natural world: complex, myste- ...f bursting through the categories of knowledge we have con- ...t.' This 'bursting through' is just what happens when Lang's ...instruct him, forcing him to revise his life. *Learning Sickness* is ...educated in the difficult school of illness, and it points to the ...at may be found there."

...hor of *Heaven's Coast* and *Firebird*

...general, and inflammatory bowel disease in particular, have ...Lang's *Learning Sickness*. It is a voice of wisdom, of courage, of ...ion. You will be touched and inspired by a powerful story told

...managing partner of Winston Partners

...a beautifully written, frank account of one man's struggle to ...the chronic illness that altered every aspect of his life. This is ...rmative book that will be of value to all patients, whether they ...nmatory bowel disease for many years or have just been diag-

...e, President and CEO, Crohn's and Colitis Foundation of America (CCFA)

...ective first person narrative of the journey of a young profes- ...ess and appreciation of life after being diagnosed with Crohn's ...he spirit of Anatole Broyard's *Intoxicated by My Illness*, but ...out dying as an end-point, Lang writes about learning how to ...ven those who are not living with chronic illness will benefit ...to live each and every day. Highly recommended for medical ...eople alike."

...den, Ph.D., Professor and Director of Medical Education, Department of ...opmental Biology, Vanderbilt University Medical School

...e than a brilliant description of illness; it is an articulation of ...ecovery. Honest, insightful, often funny, this is a book that ...e the sheer animal pleasure of being alive. Read it and experi- ...ice."

...author of *Return of the Osprey*

...st, this book is not merely the story of a man negotiating the ...ed by Crohn's disease and the medical establishment: It is ulti- ...piritual journey, shaped by the author's commitment to come ...'d lessons taught by chronic disease."

...assistant professor of English, Assumption College

Advance Pra

"Thank you, Jim Lang, for sharin
through illness and back to health
in these pages, so wonderfully w
own early trials with Crohn's disea
chronic illness who feel they may
—Jill Sklar, author of *The First Yea*

"In his book *Learning Sickness,* Jan
standing chronic illness. His perso
to be turned away from learning
assumes the appearance of a bitt
he observes 'life pulses on.' He
miracle cure, but is actually an an
him all along. The reader will ne
hand of a child again without a r
chronic illness in its full measure
—Barbara Wolcott, Pulitzer Priz
Beach-Cleaning Machine

"As a patient with Crohn's disea
is so evident not only in Jim La
willingness to share his experie
Crohn's disease, I see Jim's boo
ers—doctors, insurers, governm
resources to patients—to unders
about having a chronic illness is
overcoming that isolation."
—Jennifer Jaff, attorney

"Written with clarity and hone
informative. But Lang is intent o
and of the individual's developm
cover a humble, daily but ultin
through—suffering."
—Reginald Gibbons, Professor
author of *Sweetbitter*

"A touching and true account o
impact it has on one's life . . . .
—Annette D'Ercole, fellow inf
child with Crohn's disease

"One of Lang's central lessons i
to recognize yourself as a perso
is larger than a meditation on (

This book explor
what true health
—Joe Kraus,

"'The human bo
textbook. It is ins
rious, and capabl
structed to conta
own body begins
a book about bei
hard-won wisdom
—Mark Doty,

"Chronic illness
found a voice in J
hope, and of inspi
by a gifted writer.
—Marvin Bus

"Learning Sickness
come to terms wi
an inspiring and i
have lived with in
nosed."
—Rodger DeF

"An honest and re
sional to self-awar
disease. Written i
instead of writing
live each day fully.
from Lang's strugg
practitioners and la
—Jeanette J. N
Cell and De

"Lang's work is m
health, family, and
makes you apprecia
ence a strong new
—David Gessn

"Eloquent and hor
specific obstacles p
mately the tale of a
to terms with the h
—Michael Lanc